Prenatal Cocaine Exposure

Scientific Considerations and Policy Implications

Suzanne L. Wenzel

Barry E. Kosofsky

John A. Harvey

Martin Y. Iguchi

Paul Steinberg

Katherine E. Watkins

Rashid Shaikh

T0159545

RAND *Drug Policy Research Center* 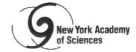 New York Academy of Sciences

This report was prepared by RAND's Drug Policy Research Center and by the New York Academy of Sciences.

ISBN: 0-8330-3001-9

Published 2001 by RAND
1700 Main Street, P.O. Box 2138, Santa Monica, CA 90407-2138
1200 South Hayes Street, Arlington, VA 22202-5050
201 North Craig Street, Suite 102, Pittsburgh, PA 15213-1516
RAND URL: http://www.rand.org/
To order RAND documents or to obtain additional information, contact Distribution Services: Telephone: (310) 451-7002; Fax: (310) 451-6915; Internet: order@rand.org

This report, a collaborative effort of the RAND Drug Policy Research Center and the New York Academy of Sciences, presents an overview of the current state of knowledge regarding the effects of cocaine on the developing brain and offers policy considerations for addressing the issues that arise from cocaine use by pregnant women. Most of the scientific research discussed in the report is derived from a 1997 New York Academy of Sciences conference on "Cocaine: Effects on the Developing Brain," the proceedings of which have been published as Volume 846 of the *Annals of the New York Academy of Sciences*. The conference was co-sponsored by the Allegheny University of the Health Sciences (now called MCP Hahnemann University) and the National Institutes of Health. The policy implications discussed here are based on material presented at this conference and on investigations conducted by researchers at RAND under the leadership of Dr. Gail Zellman.

THE RAND DRUG POLICY RESEARCH CENTER

The Drug Policy Research Center, a joint endeavor of RAND Criminal Justice and RAND Health, was established in 1989 to conduct the empirical research, policy analysis, and outreach needed to help community leaders and public officials develop more effective strategies for dealing with drug problems. The Center builds on a long tradition of RAND research characterized by an interdisciplinary, empirical approach to public policy issues and rigorous standards of quality, objectivity, and independence. The Ford Foundation and other foundations, as well as government agencies, corporations, and individuals, support the Center. Dr. Audrey Burnam and Dr. Martin Iguchi codirect the Drug Policy Research Center.

THE NEW YORK ACADEMY OF SCIENCES

Founded in 1817, the New York Academy of Sciences is the third oldest scientific organization in America and one of New York City's oldest and most enduring cultural institutions. The Academy is an independent, nonprofit organization with more than 30,000 members in more than 160 counties united by a commitment to promoting science and technology and their essential roles in fostering social and economic development. In service to science, the Academy facilitates communication among scientists, physicians, policymakers, government officers, educators, and journalists from around the world through its interdisciplinary conferences and section meetings and diverse publications. In service to society, Academy programs draw upon the foremost experts and the most current information about advances in science and technology to inform analysis and discussion of public policy issues, to promote precollege education, and to foster the human rights of scientists. The Academy also recognizes the unique relationship between science and art, and its gallery regularly features public exhibitions and musical evenings.

CONTENTS

Prenatal exposure to drugs, including cocaine, is a significant and preventable cause of developmental disability. Almost two decades after the nation first heard stories of "crack babies," new research has shown that children exposed to cocaine before birth are at risk of learning and behavioral problems. Such problems have broad implications for education, social welfare, and criminal justice in the United States.

This report presents an overview of the current state of knowledge regarding the effects of cocaine on the developing brain and offers policy considerations for addressing the issues that arise from cocaine use by pregnant women. Most of the scientific research discussed in the report is derived from a 1997 New York Academy of Sciences conference on "Cocaine: Effects on the Developing Brain," the proceedings of which have been published as Volume 846 of the *Annals of the New York Academy of Sciences* (Harvey and Kosofsky, 1998). The policy implications discussed here are based on material presented at this conference and on investigations conducted by researchers at RAND.

The report discusses three preventive strategies: primary prevention (preventing substance use before and during pregnancy); secondary prevention (identifying pregnant women who use drugs and minimizing their drug use); and tertiary prevention (reducing the adverse consequences of substance exposure in children who were exposed *in utero*). In addition, a number of areas where more research is needed are discussed and a rationale is offered for making more resources available for women and children affected by cocaine.

PRIMARY PREVENTION

Although the problems of children exposed to cocaine *in utero* are not as severe as was once feared, some cocaine-exposed infants do suffer subtle neurological damage and later have learning and behavioral problems. A number of research studies have reported that children prenatally exposed to cocaine experience reduced fetal growth (e.g., small head size), lower IQ levels, and neurobehavioral symptoms (e.g., attention difficulties). On entering school, many cocaine-exposed children have difficulty in regulating behaviors (e.g., they exhibit inattentiveness and impulsiveness), and this has an adverse effect on academic success and on adaptability and functioning later in life.

Primary prevention—avoiding cocaine and other drug use before and during pregnancy—remains the best approach to preventing exposure. It is important that women who are pregnant or who are at risk for pregnancy be educated about the potential dangers to the fetus from all forms and levels of prenatal exposure to harmful substances, including alcohol, cigarettes, and marijuana, as well as cocaine.

SECONDARY PREVENTION

Many pregnant women receive inadequate prenatal care or none at all, and many physicians are ill prepared to identify substance abuse in pregnant women or to refer the women to treatment. Consequently, most cases of substance abuse among pregnant women come to light at the time of childbirth. Secondary prevention strategies refer to the identification by health-care providers of cocaine use by pregnant women and steps taken to safeguard the health and welfare of the mother as well as to minimize effects of the drug on the fetus. Secondary prevention can have an important impact during pregnancy.

When physicians are trained in exposure-detection techniques and are confident in their ability to manage maternal and prenatal substance exposure, the potential for minimizing drug use and subsequent damage to the fetus is increased. A RAND survey of obstetricians and pediatricians revealed that training had a significant impact on a physician's ability to detect and follow up on signs and symptoms of substance use.

Although many states have enacted legislation requiring physicians to report cases of drug abuse during pregnancy, one-fifth of the physicians surveyed in the RAND study were not aware of their state's or their hospital's policies regarding reporting and follow-up procedures. Physicians' awareness of institutional and legal requirements was found to be associated with a greater propensity on the part of physicians to report drug abuse.

Most state-mandated policies and hospital protocols rely on the physician to take specific actions. Therefore, physicians should be involved in the design and implementation of such policies, and the protocols should be responsive to physicians' ethical and personal concerns. Additionally, direct incentives should be provided to hospitals to design protocols for substance-abuse reporting by health-care providers. Finally, substance-abuse information should be used only for helping the woman and the fetus; it should not be used for prosecution of the woman. The goal of detection and reporting policies should be to provide counseling, education, and treatment, not to punish or stigmatize.

Secondary prevention strategies aimed at health-care providers should include (1) education and training in substance-abuse detection techniques, (2) education about state and institutional protocols for reporting prenatal substance exposure, and (3) involvement of physicians in designing and implementing the protocols.

TERTIARY PREVENTION

Although research has shown that *in utero* cocaine exposure leads to subtle neurological changes and is associated with learning and behavioral problems that manifest in childhood, cocaine exposure does not affect all children equally, and a number of environmental (e.g., home environment), biological (e.g., adaptability), and other factors (e.g., malnutrition) also have an impact on the children's outcomes. In addition, very little is known about the long-term effects of prenatal cocaine exposure. More research is required to enable health-care providers to identify at-risk children, to understand the nature of their deficits, and to intervene on their behalf.

RESEARCH ON THE EFFECTS OF COCAINE ON THE DEVELOPING BRAIN

This report discusses three major areas where more research is needed: (1) the specific action of cocaine on the developing brain and its manifestations in infants and children; (2) the role of environmental and other factors; and (3) community and educational interventions.

Specific Action of Cocaine on the Developing Brain and Subsequent Manifestations

Animal and human studies indicate that gestational exposure to cocaine interferes with the growth and development of the brain, but the precise way in which these structural changes cause cognitive or behavioral deficits is not yet clear. Moreover, not all children exposed to cocaine *in utero* suffer neurobehavioral injuries, and those who are affected exhibit a range of neurobehavioral effects. It appears that the brain has compensatory mechanisms to provide relief from the effects of prenatal exposure to cocaine, but these mechanisms have their limits and may break down under stress in some children.

The general IQ and neurobehavioral tests now used to assess children who were prenatally exposed to cocaine may not be appropriate. The identification of specific clinical markers for neural injury from prenatal cocaine exposure would help to determine which populations of children are at risk and would aid in the development of appropriate interventions.

More research is needed on (1) the neurobiologic specificity of cocaine's action in the developing human brain; (2) the identification of compensatory mechanisms in the developing brain that may overcome effects of cocaine-induced changes; (3) the relationship between cocaine exposure and limits of adaptability in response to stress; (4) the identification of clinical markers for prenatal cocaine exposure that can be used in early infancy; and (5) the development, refinement, and validation of tests that are specific for the neurological, behavioral, and cognitive impacts of cocaine in children.

The Role of the Environment and Other Factors

The range of outcomes reported in cocaine-exposed children may result partly from factors other than, or interactive with, cocaine exposure *in utero*. These factors include multiple drug abuse, smoking, malnutrition, and unstable and stressful family life. Several studies are currently attempting to tease out the relative contribution of the various factors, but much more work needs to be done.

Community and Educational Interventions for At-Risk Children

There is relatively little information on community-based interventions directed at children prenatally exposed to cocaine. Because the effects of prenatal cocaine exposure go beyond cognitive and medical needs and children prenatally exposed to cocaine very often have a host of other difficulties, it is critical that health-care providers work in tandem with other service providers. Community-based research should be undertaken to determine the best treatment and education interventions for dealing with the effects of prenatal cocaine exposure, and providers who work with children who have been prenatally exposed to cocaine should be educated about and aware of all community resources and services.

RESOURCES FOR WOMEN AND CHILDREN: AN URGENT NEED

The effects of cocaine on the developing fetus are actively being investigated, but the results of such research are not likely to be available for some time. In the interim, sufficient warning signs exist to warrant immediate interventions at multiple levels to help cocaine-using women and their children. Such interventions are needed to reduce both the adverse health outcomes and the social costs of prenatal substance exposure.

Helping children requires a community response that involves not only health-care professionals but also a broad array of interconnected service providers who can offer the necessary diversity of expertise.

Substance-abusing women of childbearing age need every opportunity to receive treatment and other services that will help them make reasonable decisions related to their pregnancy and to caring for their children. These services should be comprehensive, also addressing problems such as poverty, homelessness, and psychiatric disorders, which often accompany cocaine use.

Resources for women and children are urgently needed. It is recommended that (1) comprehensive substance-abuse treatment services be made available to women of childbearing age; (2) treatment programs for children prenatally exposed to cocaine be implemented and operated within a framework that considers the children's home environments and offers a community response in which all service providers work together; and (3) training in serving mothers and their cocaine-exposed children be mandated for all relevant health-care providers in the community.

Chapter One

INTRODUCTION

Prenatal exposure of children to both licit drugs (such as alcohol and cigarettes) and illicit drugs (such as cocaine, marijuana, and opiates) is a substantial problem in the United States. Each year, an estimated 757,000 pregnant women use alcohol, and 820,000 smoke cigarettes. Approximately 221,000 pregnant women use an illicit drug at least once during their pregnancy, and one in five of those women (44,000) smokes crack cocaine. Moreover, approximately 32 percent of women who use one illicit drug during pregnancy also use both alcohol and cigarettes.

From these estimates, it is reasonable to assume that more than 1 million children each year are exposed to licit or illicit substances during gestation (Chasnoff, 1998). These figures, derived from the National Pregnancy and Health Survey (National Institute on Drug Abuse, 1996), are based on women's self-reports of use and therefore are likely to underestimate the extent of prenatal substance exposure.

Even these conservative estimates make it clear that prenatal exposure to drugs, both licit and illicit, is a significant and preventable cause of developmental disability. Moreover, drug abuse is prevalent in all social and economic strata, and the cost of drug treatment and rehabilitation is borne in one form or another by society as a whole.

COCAINE USE BY PREGNANT WOMEN

According to the National Household Survey on Drug Abuse, 3.4 percent (95 percent confidence interval = 2.6 percent – 4.5 percent) of the women in the United States between the ages of 18 and 25 reported using cocaine during 1998 (Substance Abuse and Mental Health Services Administration, 1999). Although it is difficult to quantify the use of cocaine by pregnant women, one study found it to be the most prevalent drug to which foster-care children had been exposed before birth. Between 1986 and 1991, the two years studied, the exposure incidence jumped from 17 percent to 55 percent of young foster-care children. The study also found that about 25 percent of the children in the 1991 study had been exposed *in utero* to more than one substance (U.S. General Accounting Office, 1997).

Cocaine is water-soluble; it can be taken orally or intravenously, or vapors of the freebase alkaloid known as crack cocaine can be inhaled. Cocaine administered by any of these routes has a strong effect on the nervous system (Chiriboga, 1998; Koren et al., 1998). It works by blocking the reuptake, or reabsorption, of certain chemicals called neurotransmitters which serve as messengers in the transmission of signals throughout the nervous system. In particular, the drug interferes with the reuptake of three neurotransmitters: dopamine, serotonin, and norepinephrine. These neurotransmitters form the monoaminergic system, which directly affects communication in other systems throughout the brain. In addition, enzymes in the body convert cocaine to its metabolites, which may have independent toxic effects on the nervous system.

Cocaine and its metabolites pass readily through the placenta to the fetus (Chiriboga, 1998), but the precise way in which cocaine affects the developing fetus is not fully understood. The neurotransmitters that make up the monoaminergic systems also have a maturational function in determining how tissues, including the brain, mature during development. To the extent that these maturational signals are interrupted by cocaine use, other deficits in the fetus may also occur.

PRENATAL COCAINE EXPOSURE AND POLICY INTERVENTIONS

Most interventions to address the problem of prenatal substance exposure have been directed at preventing the problem in the first place. For example, significant resources have been devoted to educating women about the dangers of smoking and drinking during pregnancy. These educational efforts have been supplemented with legislation mandating warning labels on cigarettes and alcohol. Steps have also been taken to educate women about the dangers of using illicit substances such as cocaine during pregnancy. The nation has made a strong effort to reduce the use of illicit drugs by making their trade, sale, and use a criminal offense (Rydell and Everingham, 1994).

Unfortunately, such prevention efforts have not been completely successful, and as the statistics above illustrate, approximately 1 million babies each year are affected by prenatal substance use. Little public attention was given to women with substance-abuse problems until the late 1970s, when the impact of prenatal alcohol exposure on children received wide publicity. Stories in the popular press in the late 1980s provided pessimistic descriptions of children exposed to cocaine *in utero*, dubbed "crack babies," suggesting that they were significantly and permanently disabled (Cosden et al., 1997; Elliott and Coker, 1991; Richardson, 1998). Follow-up studies have shown that the deficits are more subtle than initially feared; however, some of the children do have a host of learning and behavioral problems (Harvey and Kosofsky, 1998). Thus, policy approaches must be developed that address not only prevention of substance use during pregnancy but also the concerns of children born with drug-associated problems.

Drawing from the field of public health, the policy approaches that address prenatal substance exposure may be conceptualized as a spectrum of interventions ranging from primary prevention to secondary and tertiary prevention. Primary prevention, aimed at preventing the initial occurrence of a problem, refers to preventing substance use during pregnancy or avoiding pregnancy while using substances. Secondary prevention, aimed at minimization of problems when a risk factor already exists, refers to identifying pregnant women who are abusing drugs and minimizing their use of such substances. Tertiary prevention, aimed at minimizing the postexposure consequences of a problem, refers to reducing the adverse consequences of substance exposure in infants and children who have been exposed *in utero*. Given the medical, psychological, and social complexities of drug use, it appears likely that a combination of strategies focusing on all aspects of prevention will be needed to combat the full range of problems related to prenatal drug exposure.

Options for intervention include treatment and research in addition to educational and legislative strategies. These four approaches are generally applied with different emphases. For example, educational interventions for primary prevention would focus on women of childbearing age or on other members of the community who have an effect on these women's behavior. Educational intervention for secondary prevention would focus on health-care providers such as gynecologists, obstetricians, and other professionals who deal with pregnant women and their developing fetuses. And in tertiary prevention, the focus of educational interventions would be on pediatricians, educators, child-care workers, and others who provide social services to the affected children.

These options are interrelated and interdependent. Basic research interventions drive and inform education, treatment, and legislative interventions. For example, without substantial research showing the adverse effects of cigarette smoking on the fetus during pregnancy, there would no basis for pursuing educational efforts to discourage mothers from smoking or for mandating warning labels on cigarette packages regarding the connection between smoking and pregnancy. Basic research is also the driving force behind treatment interventions—the nicotine patch was developed through research on the psychopharmacology of smoking.

This report focuses on cocaine, but it is nearly impossible to separate the impact of cocaine on a fetus from other factors—including poverty and multiple drug use—that are often associated with cocaine use and that affect the outcomes of exposed children. For this reason, whenever possible, we discuss policy recommendations concerning cocaine and its associated issues within the context of the environment and other influencing factors.

FOCUS AND STRUCTURE OF THE REPORT

This report discusses prenatal exposure to cocaine, options for intervention, and areas that deserve more research and additional resources. A particular focus is prevention strategies in areas to which, until recently, only limited attention has been paid. Our discussion is informed by recent animal and clinical research in biomedical and social sciences, results of which were presented at a conference on "Cocaine: Effects on the Developing Brain," held under the auspices of the New York Academy of Sciences (NYAS) (Harvey and Kosofsky, 1998).

This report also discusses the social science research of Gail Zellman and colleagues from RAND regarding the ways in which the health-care system deals with prenatal substance exposure (Zellman, 1997; Zellman and Bell, 1990; Zellman et al., 1992, 1993, 1997). These investigators, in a study sponsored by the National Institute on Drug Abuse, performed the first national survey of hospital and physician response to prenatal substance exposure. They received completed surveys from more than 1,000 obstetricians and pediatricians who treat newborns. They also surveyed nurse managers and administrators at the hospitals where those physicians practiced to obtain information on nurses' responses and hospital protocols relating to prenatal substance exposure.

Although many questions concerning prenatal cocaine exposure remain unanswered, the information available to date provides a sound foundation for a series of policy interventions aimed at addressing the problem. It is our hope that this report will provide general guidance to decisionmakers seeking to implement these policy interventions.

Chapter Two

POLICY INTERVENTIONS FOR PREVENTION

POLICY INTERVENTIONS FOR PRIMARY PREVENTION

Primary prevention focuses on informing women of childbearing age about the dangers of prenatal cocaine exposure and educating them to abstain from cocaine use during pregnancy or to avoid pregnancy during substance use. A cocaine-exposed infant may look normal at birth, but data from several preclinical and clinical studies indicate that he or she may have experienced neurological damage that will have adverse effects later in life.

Effects of Prenatal Cocaine Exposure

The effects of prenatal cocaine exposure are the subject of a number of ongoing studies; interim results from several such studies were presented at the NYAS conference. In the Maternal Health Practices and Child Development Project, Richardson (1998) found a subtle pattern of central-nervous-system effects related to cocaine in the children of a group of 271 women who used cocaine during pregnancy. Children at age 3 who had been exposed to cocaine during the first trimester of pregnancy had smaller head circumferences and lower scores on standardized IQ tests, were fussier, and exhibited more difficult behavior than children not exposed to cocaine. Such effects were more difficult to detect at ages younger than 3.

Similarly, Mayes et al. (1998) performed a longitudinal study of 377 infants prenatally exposed to cocaine. They examined the neuro-physiological and emotional reactions of the children to a series of "novel stimuli" at 12, 18, and 54 months and concluded that the prenatally exposed children demonstrated significantly greater behavioral/performance disruptions than did children who had not been exposed to cocaine. These responses were described as "overarousal" or "overstimulation" and were incongruent with the orientation-focused attention required by the novel stimuli; such abnormalities are thought to impede learning and memory formation.

In a longitudinal, prospective study, Chasnoff et al. (1998) examined outcomes for 95 4- to 6-year-old children who had experienced prenatal cocaine exposure and 75 matched, nonexposed children. The mothers of the exposed children were all heavy cocaine users who had received comprehensive prenatal care and voluntarily enrolled in an intensive treatment program; most of them also used other substances such as alcohol, tobacco, and marijuana. Prenatal cocaine exposure did not have a direct effect on the cognitive abilities of the children; however, the exposure affected their behavioral characteristics at 4 to 6 years of age. A significant number of the exposed children showed measurably elevated levels of aggression, delinquent behavior, attention problems, and social difficulties.

Educating Cocaine Users About the Dangers of Prenatal Cocaine Exposure

Although these studies are preliminary and ongoing, they strongly indicate that prenatal cocaine exposure can adversely affect the developing fetus. The effects of cocaine exposure appear to be persistent and to have an adverse impact on the child's ability to acquire knowledge and to adapt. It is therefore important that women who are pregnant or at risk of pregnancy be educated about the potential danger to the fetus from all forms and levels of exposure to cocaine and other harmful substances, including alcohol and cigarettes.

POLICY INTERVENTIONS FOR SECONDARY PREVENTION

Secondary prevention focuses primarily on health-care providers and is concerned with identifying pregnant drug users and minimizing their use of drugs through educational, treatment, research, and regulatory interventions. Social science research, along with data from preclinical and clinical investigations, supports such interventions.

Relatively little attention has been paid to early detection of substance use during pregnancy (Zellman et al., 1992, 1997). Many pregnant women receive little or inadequate prenatal care, and many physicians are ill prepared to identify substance abuse in pregnant women or to refer them to treatment. Consequently, the majority of prenatal substance exposure cases are identified only at the time of birth, when the mother or neonate presents with signs or symptoms consistent with drug use.

Response by health-care providers to identification of drug use during pregnancy varies considerably across the states and is affected by a number of factors, including whether specific legislation exists, whether exposure is covered under child-abuse-reporting mandates, whether a public-health model (e.g., education, treatment, counseling) or a punitive model (criminal sanctions against the mother) is followed, and the specific role played by physicians in addressing substance use by pregnant patients (Chavkin et al., 1998a, 1998b; Zellman et al., 1997). As of 1997, of the 50 states and the District of Columbia, 20 had taken no specific legal action regarding prenatal substance exposure; another 20 mandated or supported less-punitive responses such as counseling or toxicology screens during pregnancy by providers or facilities; and the remaining 11 mandated child-abuse reporting when a child-serving professional suspects exposure (Zellman et al., 1997).

Women may be particularly motivated to change their behavior during pregnancy, which makes public-health-oriented, prebirth interventions such as detection and education by health-care providers an attractive approach. The effectiveness of health-care providers in reducing substance abuse during pregnancy is supported by limited research indicating that, for example, physicians' advice regarding smoking cessation during pregnancy is often effective (Ockene, 1987; Pederson, 1982).

Training Health-Care Providers to Detect Substance Use

A fundamental component of prebirth intervention is substance-use detection by health-care providers. Zellman et al. have investigated the health-care system's response to prenatal substance exposure in a legislative context (Zellman, 1997; Zellman and Bell, 1990; Zellman et al., 1992, 1993, 1997). In 1995, they mailed surveys nationwide to 3,200 practicing physicians whose primary specialty was identified as obstetrics or pediatrics in the AMA Masterfile of Physicians, which lists all physicians by primary practice specialty. Twenty-one percent of the sampled obstetricians and pediatricians indicated that they were not currently delivering infants or examining newborns less than 24 hours of age; these physicians were excluded from the study. The response rate among the remaining physicians was 63 percent. The results of the survey include the following:

- 27 percent of the respondents reported never suspecting prenatal substance exposure.

- More than 70 percent reported suspecting prenatal substance exposure at some time and taking action themselves or initiating an action through another person. Their actions included performing urine toxicology screens, taking a substance-abuse history, discussing treatment options with the mother, discussing their concern with the mother's primary-care physician, and reporting the mother to a social worker at the hospital.

- Among the physicians who reported having suspected prenatal substance exposure at some time, 82 percent said that they always responded to their suspicion in some way. The remainder did not consistently respond to their suspicion, giving a lack of sufficient evidence that substance abuse had occurred as the most common reason for not responding.

- 80 percent of the obstetricians reported that they had delivered at least one baby who turned out to have been exposed during pregnancy, although the physicians had not suspected exposure.

The obstetricians and pediatricians who suspected prenatal substance exposure at some time and those who never suspected it could be easily distinguished by the amount of formal training in prenatal exposure they had received and their confidence in their ability to manage substance-using women during pregnancy or substance-exposed infants (Zellman et al., 1997).

These findings suggest that levels of vigilance and response could be increased by providing more training to physicians; more training would also make physicians more confident in their ability to identify the problem and respond to it.

Educating Health-Care Providers About the Importance of Prenatal-Substance-Use Policies

In their survey of obstetricians and pediatricians, Zellman et al. (1997) also investigated the physicians' awareness of workplace protocols and state reporting requirements regarding prenatal substance exposure. They found that

- 51 percent of the eligible physicians in the survey reported that there is a protocol governing prenatal substance exposure in the hospital where they perform the most deliveries or see the most newborns.

- Just over one-fourth (27 percent) reported that there is no protocol at their hospital, and, notably, one-fifth (21 percent) did not know whether such a protocol exists in their hospital.

The investigators also provided the physicians with a list of maternal and neonatal signs and symptoms and asked them about their knowledge of state mandates: "Are MDs in your state legally obligated to make a child maltreatment report when their suspicions of prenatal substance exposure are based on [insert sign or symptom]?" They found that

- More than 40 percent of all respondents did not know whether a child-maltreatment report was necessary under their state's law in response to the given set of signs and symptoms.

This lack of knowledge among two-fifths of the physicians surveyed about institutional and legal requirements is important given the researchers' findings that physician awareness is associated with the propensity to report exposure. That is, knowledge of the existence of hospital protocols on maternal substance use or prenatal substance exposure was associated with a greater likelihood of physician response when they suspected exposure. Among physicians who reported some knowledge of their state's reporting requirements, those residing in mandatory-reporting states were the most likely to believe that suspicion of exposure requires a report of child maltreatment (Zellman et al., 1997).

Frequently, the message that laws and policies governing prenatal substance exposure exist does not reach physicians, who are in the best position to detect and respond to exposure (Zellman et al., 1997). However, research indicates that laws and policies can influence physician behavior when the physicians receive the message and when the mandated response is clear (e.g., the requirement of a child-maltreatment report) (Zellman et al., 1997).

Involving Health-Care Providers in Designing Hospital Protocols

Most legislative approaches that address prenatal substance exposure rely heavily on physicians to detect substance use and take action (Zellman et al., 1997). Physicians' ability to do so, however, is constrained by several factors. Many physicians surveyed by Zellman et al. described concerns about disruption in care as an important reason for deciding not to act on suspicion of prenatal substance exposure. The reporting systems also add to physicians' work and costs by requiring additional time. The child-abuse-reporting literature suggests that the costs are often perceived to outweigh the benefits, and consequently, compliance rates are low (Zellman and Bell, 1990).

Hospital protocols requiring reporting of suspected substance abuse can be made more effective by involving physicians in developing and implementing them and by ensuring that physicians' ethical and professional concerns are addressed. In addition, policies aimed at physician behavior can be complemented by the assignment of certain responsibilities to the hospital where care is administered. Finally, medical personnel other than physicians can also play an important role in detection and referral and should be included in the process of developing or implementing protocols. Nurses, in particular, are well positioned to alert physicians to a mother's or neonate's presenting symptoms.

Providing Incentives to Hospitals to Design Reporting Protocols

Zellman et al. (1997) showed that physicians are more likely to respond to their suspicions of maternal substance use when they believe that their hospital has a protocol for responding to prenatal substance exposure. State legislators should establish direct incentives for hospitals to implement protocols requiring substance-use screening of all women in a routine and nonstigmatizing fashion.

Avoiding Penalties for Mothers of Prenatally Exposed Children

Although the dilemma of balancing the welfare of the child with the rights and responsibilities of the mother is far from resolved, punitive legislation is a prominent component of the U.S. response to the public-health threat of prenatal substance exposure. The number of states in which cocaine-using mothers were criminally prosecuted increased from 22 to 34 between 1992 to 1995 (Chavkin et al., 1998a). Policies that punish substance-using women typically do not provide them with treatment options (Chavkin et al., 1998b). Citing a lack of evidence that punitive approaches are effective, a consensus panel on pregnant substance-using women, organized by the Center for Substance Abuse Treatment, advised against the criminal prosecution of these women (Center for Substance Abuse Treatment, 1993b). From a public-health perspective, criminal prosecution does not protect the health of the woman or that of the fetus and plays no role in secondary-prevention strategies. Substance-abuse detection and reporting policies should be aimed at providing counseling, education, and treatment, not punishment or stigmatization of the woman.

POLICY INTERVENTIONS FOR TERTIARY PREVENTION

Tertiary prevention consists of steps taken to reduce the adverse outcomes of cocaine exposure in infants and children. Ameliorating any damage and promoting a healthy home environment are critical for prenatally exposed infants. New insights gained through research into cocaine's action on the brain not only make it possible to intervene more effectively on behalf of at-risk children but can also be used to strengthen support for prevention strategies that, from a public-health perspective, are in the best interests of both the child and society.

Neonatal outcomes associated with prenatal cocaine exposure include reduced fetal growth (e.g., low birth weight, intrauterine growth retardation, and small head size), decreases in IQ levels,[1] and the development of neurobehavioral symptoms, such as problems in regulating excitability and attention. Cocaine appears to alter fetal brain development and to be associated with lasting changes in brain structure and function that have subtle but important implications for learning and behavior in some exposed individuals. A pivotal conclusion emerging from the NYAS conference is that as some of the prenatally exposed children enter school, they experience difficulty in regulating behaviors (e.g., attention and impulsiveness) that are critical to their academic success, and this bodes poorly for adaptability and functioning in later life.

There are, however, many critical gaps in our knowledge of the effects of prenatal cocaine exposure. For example, the long-term effects of prenatal substance exposure are poorly understood. While some neurological and cognitive effects may be self-limiting and may resolve by childhood, there is strong evidence for a lasting problem of inattention (Chiriboga, 1998). However, some of the cognitive deficits may be associated with only the highest cocaine exposures, which result in a reduction in brain growth and smaller head size. More research is needed to develop greater understanding of the long-term effects (direct and indirect) of prenatal substance exposure; such research would provide the foundation for identification and intervention to help children who are at risk.

---

[1]The implications of even small shifts in IQ scores are significant (Lester, 1998). A shift of five points, for example, results in very little change in the largest area under the bell curve depicting the normal distribution of IQ scores, where most of the population lies. However, in the tails, where extreme IQ scores lie, a five-point shift would result in a loss of two-thirds of the people who are in the highest IQ bracket and would triple the number of people with very low IQs.

Chapter Three

AREAS IN WHICH MORE RESEARCH ON THE EFFECTS OF COCAINE IS NEEDED

This chapter summarizes three areas in which research can increase understanding of effects of prenatal cocaine exposure: (1) the specific action of cocaine on the developing brain and its manifestation in infants and children, (2) the role of environmental factors that either act alone or interact with cocaine, and (3) community and educational interventions required for cocaine-exposed infants and children.

THE NEUROBIOLOGIC SPECIFICITY OF COCAINE ACTION

Mechanisms of Action of Cocaine

As noted earlier, the precise mechanism of action of cocaine is not well understood. In addition to its influence on neurotransmitters, cocaine can affect the developing brain by inducing hypoxia (oxygen deprivation) through direct toxicity; it can also induce cortical dysgenesis (impaired development of the cortex) by altering aminergic signals required for normal brain growth (Chiriboga, 1998).

Understanding the precise effects of cocaine requires elucidation of the mechanisms of the drug's absorption, distribution, metabolism, and excretion; molecular and cellular alterations following exposure; effects on specific neurochemical systems in the brain; and the interaction or combination of cocaine with other drugs and insults such as malnutrition.

Both animal and human studies support the hypothesis that gestational exposure to cocaine affects the way the fetal brain grows and develops (Chiriboga, 1998; Ferriero, 1998 [Table 1]; Kosofsky and Wilkins, 1998; Mayes et al., 1998; Nassogne, Evrard, and Courtoy, 1998; Romano and Harvey, 1998). There is also a dose-response relationship between cocaine exposure and head size (Kosofsky and Wilkins, 1998), although the timing and specificity of the gestational exposure on development and behavior remain to be defined (Ferriero, 1998; Mayes et al., 1998).

It is not clear how the structural changes apparent in the brains of cocaine-exposed animals and humans cause cognitive and/or behavioral deficits. For example, cocaine-exposed infants have lower mean head circumferences than do unexposed infants, and microcephaly (small head size) predicts poor cognitive performance; however, the way in which microcephaly leads to poor performance is not understood (Chiriboga, 1998; Nassogne et al., 1998).

Mayes et al. (1998) present three plausible links between prenatal cocaine exposure and the mechanisms affecting cognition and behavior, specifically, arousal and attention regulation in infants and preschool-age children. These links may be attributable to the association of prenatal cocaine exposure with (1) alterations in the development and function of the monoaminergic systems, (2) alterations in brain structures underlying the response to stress (the brain systems that secrete hormones during stressful events such as disease and injury are important for recovery), and (3) alterations in other brain systems that mediate regulation of arousal (Mayes et al., 1998).

Animal models have helped to elucidate some of the relationships between brain structure and neurobehavioral function. For example, cocaine-exposed rabbits display abnormal structural and neurochemical development of the anterior cingulate cortex, a region of the brain known to be involved in associative learning, attentional processes, and motor function (Romano and Harvey, 1998). Cocaine-exposed rabbits demonstrate impairments in motor function, associative learning, and discrimination learning, which Romano and Harvey (1998) interpret as a consequence of deficits in attentional processes caused by the abnormalities within the damaged anterior cingulate cortex.

Thus, although animal and human studies indicate that gestational exposure to cocaine affects the growth and development of the brain, it is not yet clear how the structural changes in the brain cause cognitive or behavioral deficits. Preclinical and clinical research is needed gain a better understanding of the neurobiologic specificity of cocaine's action in the developing human brain.

Compensatory Mechanisms in the Developing Brain

One of the conundrums in studies of children prenatally exposed to cocaine is that although some of them suffer neurobehavioral injuries (Chasnoff et al., 1998; Lester, 1998), others with similar exposure do not. One conference attendee noted, "Not every child exposed to cocaine demonstrates brain growth retardation, inattention, cognitive impairments, or language delay. Even those children with a significant cocaine exposure and evidence of developmental compromise may not demonstrate all of these deficits" (see Kosofsky and Wilkins, 1998). Understanding how some children compensate for the effects of cocaine exposure is therefore very important.

The dose of cocaine that the fetus is exposed to will influence the outcome in the infant and child. As in the case of fetuses exposed to alcohol, there appears to be a relationship between higher levels of maternal cocaine use and greater incidence and severity of deficits in the exposed infants and children (Delaney-Black et al., 1998; Richardson, 1998). However, genetic and environmental factors are also likely to influence the incidence and severity of intrauterine cocaine exposure, and there has as yet been no demonstration of a lower limit (threshold) of drug exposure known to be safe, nor is sufficient information available to establish the dose-response relationship for the amount of maternal cocaine use and outcome.

Animal models of brain development suggest that the developing nervous system is remarkably plastic (Spear et al., 1998). However, while the developing brain may use compensatory processes to overcome the effects of early drug exposure, such neural compensation may have a cost: It may cause a decrease in the adaptability of the animal when stressed. A number of studies substantiate this argument. Dr. Theodore Slotkin, a conference participant, noted, "There may be sufficient adaptations to normalize the essential behaviors that you need to survive as a human being, but it may be adaptability that's compromised" (Harvey and Kosofsky, 1998, p. 153).

Thus, more research is needed to understand the specific mechanisms of compensation and their location and timing. Particularly valuable will be research to identify specific "recoverable deficits" so that treatments and interventions can be devised that promote compensation and recovery for cocaine-exposed children.

Adaptability in Stressful Situations

The relief provided by compensatory mechanisms has limits, and the mechanisms can break down under stress. Several animal studies demonstrate that cocaine-exposed offspring differ from control animals in their behavioral response to stressful and environmentally challenging situations (Spear et al., 1998). When confronted with stressful situations, for example, normal adult rats typically exhibit increased immobility, whereas adult rats that were exposed to cocaine *in utero* show much less of the immobility response. Cocaine-exposed rats are hyperresponsive in stressful situations, exhibiting excessive fearfulness and frantic behavior (Church et al., 1998).

In clinical populations, infants and preschool-age children exposed to cocaine *in utero* exhibit a low threshold for activating their "stress circuits" when confronted with novel challenges (Mayes et al., 1998); thus, they may be particularly vulnerable to the detrimental effects of stressful environmental conditions. Further, cocaine-exposed children appear to have a pattern of altered stress response that manifests itself by blunting the usual patterns of increased arousal in stressful situations. As a result, cocaine-exposed children need more stimulation to reach optimal states of arousal for responsiveness; at the same time, they can quickly become overaroused, inattentive, and poorly responsive. In other words, while they require more stimulation to increase arousal and attention, they modulate higher states of arousal less well (Mayes et al., 1998). Additional research is needed to discern the relationship between cocaine exposure and limits of adaptability in response to stress.

Clinical Markers of Brain Injury

Clinical markers of neural injury caused by prenatal cocaine exposure would help to identify populations of at-risk children and would facilitate the development of appropriate interventions. The available clinical markers, such as impaired brain growth, hypertonia (muscle stiffness), and impairment of cognitive function, are neither sensitive nor specific because they may also occur in alcohol- or opiate-exposed or malnourished children (see above). However, in the presence of evidence of prenatal cocaine exposure, such markers can help identify a child at potential risk and can suggest specific interventions for treating the deficits. But care must be exercised not to stigmatize such infants or their mothers.

Another important question relates to whether psychopharmacologic interventions may be effective for exposed children who demonstrate the deficits associated with exposure. For example, it is tempting to think that children who have problems with attention would benefit from the stimulants used to treat attention deficit disorders. However, it is not known whether the same neurochemical pathways are affected in the same way in both groups of children, and thus it is not known whether stimulant therapy would be appropriate. At this time, there are no systematic studies that demonstrate the benefits of any specific psychopharmacological intervention in exposed children.

Identification of specific clinical markers of neural injury from prenatal cocaine exposure would help to identify populations of exposed children at risk and would facilitate the development of appropriate interventions. Research should therefore be conducted to identify clinical markers for the exposed brain during early infancy.

Increased Sensitivity of Tests to Detect Changes in the Brain

At present, a number of tests are used to measure the effect of prenatal cocaine exposure on behavior, including standardized tests such the Connors Parent and Teacher Rating Scales; the Achenbach Child Behavior Checklist and Teacher Report Form; the Child Behavior Checklist (Parent and Teacher Forms); and the Problem Behavior

Scale (Delaney-Black et al., 1998). Although such tests are generally easy to administer and score, none of them is specific for cocaine (Chiriboga, 1998). Research-based clinical tools have also been developed to investigate the effects of cocaine exposure; for example, Mayes et al. (1998) measure the startle response, which they believe reflects arousal. Although useful, such clinical tests need to be standardized, replicated in other laboratories, and tested in larger populations of cocaine-exposed children.

A fundamental issue for all of these tests is that of whether to use a deviant or discriminant approach in assessing the effect of prenatal cocaine exposure. As discussed by Karmel (Harvey and Kosofsky, 1998, p. 341), commonly used tests such as the global IQ test follow a deviant approach, where the test population is compared to an average, "normed" population and is tested for deviation. This approach may lead to an incorrect attribution of the factors contributing to the deviance from the norm. For example, infants and children raised in impoverished environments demonstrate impaired performance on IQ tests (Lester, 1998). Because many cocaine-exposed infants are raised in impoverished environments, a comparison of performance of such children may incorrectly attribute their impairments to the cocaine exposure rather than to poverty.

A discriminant approach takes into account some of the uniqueness of the particular population being studied and can therefore be more informative. For example, comparison of the outcomes of cocaine-exposed children raised in impoverished environments with non-cocaine-exposed infants from similarly impoverished environments is much more likely to reveal meaningful differences that are specifically attributable to cocaine exposure.

THE ROLE OF THE ENVIRONMENT AND OTHER FACTORS

Because the environment and other factors influence the manifestation of cocaine-induced intrauterine insults, it is important to understand their relative contributions to the problems seen in infants and children. The wide range of outcomes reported in cocaine-exposed children may result partly from factors other than, or interactive with, cocaine. For example, the arousal response is affected by environmental factors as well as by cocaine exposure (Mayes et al., 1998). Cocaine-exposed infants are often born to families with multiple social problems, including poverty and ongoing drug/alcohol use, that lead to a less stimulating and organized home environment, which affects arousal (Koren et al., 1998, Table 1; Richardson, 1998). Cocaine-using mothers are also more likely to report a history of school-related problems, presumably prior to drug use; such problems manifest as attention deficits and learning disabilities similar to those exhibited by prenatally exposed children (Slotkin, 1998). Malnutrition during pregnancy, common among cocaine-using women, also leads to some of the same physical symptoms in their children as those observed in children prenatally exposed to cocaine (Santolaria-Fernandez et al., 1995).

Teasing out the relative contributions of prenatal cocaine exposure and environmental, genetic, and other factors has proven extremely complicated. However, some progress has been made with animal models. For example, studies in rats suggest that cocaine exposure and malnutrition may have both independent and interactive effects (Galler and Tonkiss, 1998). In these studies, prenatal cocaine exposure and malnutrition both resulted in lower birth weight and delayed physical and neurological (reflexive) development; these impairments were additive when the rats were exposed to both insults. On tests of spatial orientation, however, prenatal cocaine exposure and malnutrition resulted in different deficits, and the impairments were not additive (Galler and Tonkiss, 1998). Other studies of postnatal behavior in mice have identified the relative contributions of cocaine-induced malnutrition, which has an indirect effect on development, and the direct effect of prenatal cocaine exposure. Both malnutrition and cocaine exposure contribute to deficits in blocking (i.e., inability to ignore redundant or extraneous information), suggesting impairments in selective attention (Kosofsky and Wilkins, 1998).

Relevant animal models to assess some other behaviors and deficits, such as selective language delay, are not currently available (Kosofsky and Wilkins, 1998). Kosofsky and Wilkins have argued that "the laboratory setting is an artificial one and may not simulate the real-world challenges that tax the particular behaviors that may be compromised in cocaine-exposed offspring" (p. 257). Several ongoing research projects are now focusing on resolving such complexities.

The Toronto Adoption Study is designed to sort out the role of cocaine exposure while controlling for the postnatal environment. This study found that with prematurity and the postnatal environment controlled for, *in utero* cocaine exposure resulted in decreased postnatal brain growth, significant language delays, and a trend toward decreased IQ in 23 preschool children up to 2 years of age who had been adopted by middle- to upper-class families (Koren et al., 1998). Unfortunately, the investigators were not able to control for concurrent maternal alcohol and tobacco use.

Chasnoff et al. (1998) have examined the interaction of biological and environmental factors on the cognitive and behavioral development of children prenatally exposed to cocaine. Prenatal cocaine exposure was not found to directly affect IQ, but the home environment in families where cocaine was being used did indirectly affect IQ. However, Chasnoff et al. (1998) found that cocaine exposure had a direct adverse impact on the child's behavioral characteristics, in particular, on the child's ability to self-regulate emotional states and transitions.

Bendersky and Lewis (1998) investigated the effect of cocaine exposure on impulse control, taking into account medical factors, exposures to other substances, and caregiver behavior. They found that exposed children exhibited less impulse control than did unexposed children; however impulse control was also influenced by the caregiver's behavior, suggesting that both intrinsic and environmental factors contribute to a child's behavior.

The studies cited above demonstrate the complex influence of cocaine on a child's behavior and the influence on such behavior of myriad environmental factors. Further research is needed to identify the independent and interactive biological and environmental determinants of behavior in children exposed to cocaine *in utero*.

COMMUNITY AND EDUCATIONAL INTERVENTIONS

Treatment and Education Interventions

There is scant information available about treatment or educational interventions for children prenatally exposed to cocaine. Such children frequently experience a host of other difficulties, such as unstable families, poverty, and multiple substance abuse. As discussed above, no systematic studies have demonstrated the benefits of any specific psychopharmacological intervention for children with deficits associated with prenatal exposure to cocaine. Therefore, addressing the psychosocial problems of exposed children with support services and school- or community-based interventions is of more immediate concern. Such interventions must be closely tailored to the individual strengths, weaknesses, and specific needs of the affected child. Although no programs have been developed to meet the specific needs of cocaine-exposed children, several studies have provided evidence that well-designed intervention programs are effective.

A team of RAND investigators recently reviewed nine early-childhood intervention programs and found that each one had a favorable impact on one or more developmental, educational, economic, or health indicators measured in children at risk for a host of problems (Karoly et al., 1998). Although the analyses did not represent a complete accounting of program benefits, and most of the evaluations did not include long-term follow-up, the results showed that children in these intervention programs experienced gains in emotional or cognitive development, improvements in educational process and outcomes, and reduced levels of criminal activity. The interventions also resulted in improved parent-child relationships; increased economic self-sufficiency (initially for the parent and later for the child, through greater labor-force participation, higher income, and lower welfare usage); and improvements in health-related indicators, such as child abuse, maternal reproductive health, and maternal substance abuse. In addition, an analysis of long-term costs and benefits for three early intervention programs indicated substantial financial savings to the government (taxpayers) that far exceeded program costs.

Education of Providers About Community Resources

Because the effects of prenatal cocaine exposure go beyond the cognitive and medical realm, it is critical for health-care providers to work in tandem with other care providers (child-care providers, educators, and social workers). However, few pediatricians and obstetricians are aware of the shortage of treatment programs in most communities, and therefore few are able to advise pregnant women appropriately. Third-party payers and constrained budgets in many communities have also led to declining support for prevention and wellness. It is therefore very important that health-care providers and their support staffs be educated about resources that are available to help women and children in their community and to which those in need can be referred.

Given that dealing with children prenatally exposed to cocaine and their mothers requires a community response, the Center for Substance Abuse Treatment has recommended that training involve not only health-care professionals, but also state child-protective services, child welfare, and alcohol and drug program staff—a broad array of interconnected providers that can provide the necessary diversity of expertise (Center for Substance Abuse Treatment, 1993a). The Center for Substance Abuse Treatment has further recommended that the federal government provide training to state agency staffs, and that state agencies should in turn provide training to local programs and to all those involved in the court process. Federal funds for training would probably be required to ensure compliance with such training regulations.

Chapter Four

RESOURCES FOR WOMEN AND CHILDREN AFFECTED BY COCAINE: AN URGENT NEED

The direct effect of cocaine exposure on the fetus and the contributing role of diet, environment, and other variables on the physical and mental well-being of the child are being actively investigated. The final results of many such investigations will not be available for some time to come, but, as this report illustrates, available data point to sufficient warning signs to warrant intervention and call for multiple levels of such intervention to help the women and safeguard the children affected by prenatal cocaine exposure.

RESOURCES FOR WOMEN

All women of childbearing age should be educated about the dangers cocaine abuse poses for the fetus; women already addicted to cocaine should be treated before they become pregnant. Steps should also be taken to bolster the detection of substance abuse during pregnancy; however, the results of such detection should not lead to stigmatization or criminal prosecution of the women. The most reasonable long-term strategy is to support the mother's ability to make reasonable decisions about the care of her fetus and child and to ensure that she has the resources available to do so. Resources for cocaine-abusing women should include education to empower them to assume responsibility and to make informed and appropriate choices.

In addition, there is a compelling need for expansion of resources for treatment of women who use cocaine—a need that is now being increasingly acknowledged and investigated (Kaltenbach and Finnegan, 1998). The National Institute on Drug Abuse has developed and tested gender-specific treatment models (e.g., Rahdert, 1996), and the increased availability of resources and facilities will improve the success of the primary and secondary prevention strategies described above.

Because drug abusers often face additional problems, such as poverty, homelessness, violence, and psychiatric illness, it is important that treatment centers offer comprehensive care. The Center for Substance Abuse Treatment recommends that services be provided within a multilevel model that includes intensive outpatient, residential, and other health-care and social services (Center for Substance Abuse Treatment, 1994, 1997). Kaltenbach and Finnegan (1998) also emphasize the importance of providing comprehensive care for substance-abusing pregnant women, including high-risk obstetrical care, psychosocial services, and addiction treatment. Such care can help reduce complications associated with prenatal substance use. The researchers point out that although comprehensive services are expensive, they are ultimately cost-effective because they reduce the negative impact of prenatal cocaine exposure, lower the cost of hospital stays, and minimize foster-care and child-protective-service placements.

Despite the differing views on a number of issues pertaining to women who use cocaine during pregnancy, there is general agreement that addiction treatment is an essential component of the social response to this problem. The federal government has funded research on addiction treatment in several ways, for example, by increasing set-asides from federal substance-abuse-treatment block grants, by preferentially enrolling pregnant women for treatment, and by establishing demonstration treatment programs for drug-abusing women (Chavkin et al., 1998b).

RESOURCES FOR CHILDREN

The consequences of fetal brain injury—whether induced by prematurity, malnutrition, asphyxia, or drugs and alcohol—are critically influenced by the postnatal environment. In fact, the brain-injured infant is especially dependent on early stimulation and optimal care to promote compensatory mechanisms that can minimize the impact of prenatal insults. Early identification of infants at risk for developmental compromise and appropriate provision of services are therefore important goals.

Regardless of the types of treatment interventions recommended for prenatally exposed children, it is critical that the interventions be implemented within a caregiving environment; this is particularly important in view of the chaotic home life of many of the children. Treating problems of prenatally exposed children without addressing their environment is ineffective because a poor-quality environment strongly reinforces problem behaviors (Mayes, in Slotkin, 1998). Drug-abusing women often withdraw from interacting with their babies. Treatment plans should therefore include a specific set of caregiver/child behaviors.

As discussed above, well-designed intervention programs provide significant benefits to children at risk due to problems induced by prenatal drug exposure. Increasing the resources available for pregnant and reproductive-age women with drug problems and providing intervention services for drug-exposed infants and children can minimize the impact of a significant and preventable cause of disability in the United States. Such an investment benefits not only those women and their children, but all of American society.

Chapter Five

SOURCES FOR FURTHER INFORMATION

In addition to the many articles and books cited in the body of this report, a wide range of resources, including journal reports, books, and Internet websites, are available for readers wishing more information about programs and services for substance-using women and at-risk children. Some of these resources are listed below.

A number of federal agencies have published documents intended to facilitate service development and program implementation. These publications cover such topics as building and sustaining care systems for substance-using pregnant women and their infants (Laken and Hutchins, 1995); implementing prenatal addiction prevention and treatment programs (Center for Substance Abuse Treatment, 1996); screening for substance abuse during pregnancy, with the goal of improving care and health (Morse et al., 1997); providing guidance for primary-care physicians on delivering substance-abuse services (Sullivan and Fleming, 1997); recruiting and retaining substance-using pregnant and parenting women (Laken and Hutchins, 1996); and treating drug-exposed women and their children (Mitchell, 1993; Rahdert, 1996; Center for Substance Abuse Treatment, 1994).

Publications that focus specifically on infants and children include Olson and Burgess (1997), a discussion of early interventions; Chasnoff, Anson, and Iaukea (1998) on approaches to understanding behavior and learning; Kandall (1993) on improving learning; and a series of papers edited by Lewis and Bendersky (1995) that explore the role of toxins in development.

In addition to these print sources, Internet websites that offer a wealth of information on a variety of relevant topics and provide links to additional websites are maintained by several private organizations and government agencies. Examples include

- The American Academy of Pediatrics (http://www.aap.org) for guidelines and policy statements for providers.

- The Evan B. Donaldson Adoption Institute (http://www.adoptioninstitute.org) for information on adopting drug-exposed children.

- The Benton Foundation (http://www.connectforkids.org) for information on a wide range of subjects pertaining to child care, health, and education.

- The National Institute on Drug Abuse (http://www.nida.nih.gov).

- The Substance Abuse and Mental Health Services Administration at http://www.samhsa.gov. The Center for Substance Abuse Prevention and the Center for Substance Abuse Treatment are components of this organization.

- Administration for Children and Families (http://www.acf.dhhs.gov). This organization sponsors programs on foster care, adoption, family support, Head Start, child abuse and neglect, and child welfare.

REFERENCES

Bendersky, M., and Lewis, M. (1998). Prenatal Cocaine Exposure and Impulse Control at Two Years. In J. A. Harvey and B. E. Kosofsky (eds.), *Cocaine: Effects on the Developing Brain* (pp. 365–367). New York: The New York Academy of Sciences.

Center for Substance Abuse Treatment (1996). *From the Source: A Guide for Implementing Perinatal Addiction Prevention and Treatment Programs.* Rockville, MD: U.S. Department of Health and Human Services.

Center for Substance Abuse Treatment (1993a). *Improving Treatment for Drug-Exposed Infants.* Rockville, MD: U.S. Department of Health and Human Services.

Center for Substance Abuse Treatment (1994). *Practical Approaches in the Treatment of Women Who Use Alcohol and Other Drugs.* Rockville, MD: Department of Health and Human Services, Public Health Service.

Center for Substance Abuse Treatment (1993b). *Pregnant, Substance-Using Women.* Rockville, MD: U.S. Department of Health and Human Services.

Center for Substance Abuse Treatment (1997). *Substance Abuse Treatment and Domestic Violence.* Treatment Improvement Protocol (TIP) Series 25 (DHHS Publication SMA 97–3163). Washington, DC: U.S. Government Printing Office.

Chasnoff, I. J. (1998). Silent Violence: Is Prevention a Moral Obligation? *Pediatrics, 102,* pp. 145–148.

Chasnoff, I. J., Anson, A., Hatcher, R., Stenson, H., Iaukea, K., and Randolph, L. A. (1998). Prenatal Exposure to Cocaine and Other Drugs. Outcome at Four to Six Years. In J. A. Harvey and B. E. Kosofsky (eds.), *Cocaine: Effects on the Developing Brain* (pp. 314–328). New York: The New York Academy of Sciences.

Chasnoff I. J., Anson A. R., Iaukea, K.A.M. (1998). *Understanding the Drug-Exposed Child: Approaches to Behavior and Learning.* Chicago: Imprint Publications.

Chavkin, W., Breitbart, V., Elman, D., and Wise, P.H. (1998b). National Survey of the States: Policies and Practices Regarding Drug-Using Pregnant Women. *American Journal of Public Health, 88,* pp. 117–119.

Chavkin, W., Wise, P. H., and Elman, D. (1998a). Policies Towards Pregnancy and Addiction: Sticks Without Carrots. In J. A. Harvey and B. E. Kosofsky (eds.), *Cocaine: Effects on the Developing Brain* (pp. 335–340). New York: The New York Academy of Sciences.

Chiriboga, C. A. (1998). Neurological Correlates of Fetal Cocaine Exposure. In J. A. Harvey and B. E. Kosofsky (eds.), *Cocaine: Effects on the Developing Brain* (pp. 109–125). New York: The New York Academy of Sciences.

Church, M. W., Crossland, W. J., Holmes, P. A., Overbeck, G. W., and Tilak, J. P. (1998). Effects of Prenatal Cocaine on Hearing, Vision, Growth, and Behavior. In J. A. Harvey and B. E. Kosofsky (eds.), *Cocaine: Effects on the Developing Brain* (pp. 12–28). New York: The New York Academy of Sciences.

Cosden, M., Peerson, S., and Elliott, K. (1997). Effects of Prenatal Drug Exposure on Birth Outcomes and Early Childhood Development. *Journal of Drug Issues, 27(3),* pp. 525–539.

Delaney-Black, V., Covington, C., Templin, T., Ager, J., Martier, S., Compton, S., and Sokol, R. (1998). Prenatal Coke: What's Behind the Smoke? Prenatal Cocaine/Alcohol Exposure and School-Age Outcomes: The SCHOO-BE Experience. In J. A. Harvey and B. E. Kosofsky (eds.), *Cocaine: Effects on the Developing Brain* (pp. 277–288). New York: The New York Academy of Sciences.

Elliott, K. T., and Coker, D. R. (1991). Crack Babies: Here They Come, Ready or Not. *Journal of Instructional Psychology, 18,* pp. 60–64.

Ferriero, D. M. (1998). Moderator, Round Table 3. Specificity of Developmental Effects in the CNS. In J. A. Harvey and B. E. Kosofsky (eds.), *Cocaine: Effects on the Developing Brain* (pp. 213–221). New York: The New York Academy of Sciences.

Galler, J. R., and Tonkiss, J. (1998). The Effects of Prenatal Protein Malnutrition and Cocaine on the Development of the Rat. In J. A. Harvey and B. E. Kosofsky (eds.), *Cocaine: Effects on the Developing Brain* (pp. 29–39). New York: The New York Academy of Sciences.

Harvey, J. A., and Kosofsky, B. E. (eds.) (1998). *Cocaine: Effects on the Developing Brain.* New York: The New York Academy of Sciences. (Volume 846 of the *Annals of the New York Academy of Sciences.*)

Kaltenbach, K., and Finnegan, L. (1998). Prevention and Treatment Issues for Pregnant Cocaine-Dependent Women and Their Infants. In J. A. Harvey and B. E. Kosofsky (eds.), *Cocaine: Effects on the Developing Brain* (pp. 329–334). New York: The New York Academy of Sciences.

Kandall, S. R. (1993). *Improving Treatment for Drug-Exposed Infants.* Rockville, MD: Department of Health and Human Services.

Karoly, L. A., Greenwood, P. W., Everingham, S. S., Hoube, J., Kilburn, M. R., Rydell, C. P., Sanders, M., and Chiesa, J. (1998). *Investing in Our Children: What We Know and Don't Know About the Costs and Benefits of Early Childhood Interventions* (MR-898-TCWF). Santa Monica, CA: RAND.

Koren, G., Nulman, I., Rovet, J., Greenbaum, R., Loebstein, M., and Einarson, T. (1998). Long-Term Neurodevelopmental Risks in Children Exposed *in Utero* to Cocaine. In J. A. Harvey and B. E. Kosofsky (eds.), *Cocaine: Effects on the Developing Brain* (pp. 329–334). New York: The New York Academy of Sciences.

Kosofsky, B. E., and Wilkins, A. S. (1998). A Mouse Model of Transplacental Cocaine Exposure Clinical Implications for Exposed Infants and Children. In J. A. Harvey and B. E. Kosofsky (eds.), *Cocaine: Effects on the Developing Brain* (pp. 248–261). New York: The New York Academy of Sciences.

Laken, M.P., and Hutchins, E. (1995). *Building and Sustaining Systems of Care for Substance-Using Pregnant Women and Their Infants: Lessons Learned.* Arlington, VA: National Center for Education in Maternal and Child Health, Department of Health and Human Services.

Laken, M. P., and Hutchins, E. (1996). *Recruitment and Retention of Substance-Using Pregnant and Parenting Women: Lessons Learned.* Arlington, VA: National Center for Education in Maternal and Child Health, Department of Health and Human Services.

Lester, B. M. (1998). The Maternal Lifestyles Study. In J. A. Harvey and B. E. Kosofsky (eds.), *Cocaine: Effects on the Developing Brain* (pp. 296–305). New York: The New York Academy of Sciences.

Lewis, M., and Bendersky, M., eds. (1995). *Mothers, Babies, and Cocaine: The Role of Toxins in Development.* Hillsdale, NJ: Erlbaum.

Mayes, L. C., Grillon, C., Granger, R., and Schottenfeld, R. (1998). Regulation of Arousal and Attention in Preschool Children Exposed to Cocaine Prenatally. In J. A. Harvey and B. E. Kosofsky (eds.), *Cocaine: Effects on the Developing Brain* (pp. 126–143). New York: The New York Academy of Sciences.

Mitchell, J. L. (1993). *Pregnant, Substance-Using Women.* Treatment Improvement Protocol (TIP) number 2. Rockville, MD: U.S. Department of Health and Human Services.

Morse, B., Gehshan, S., and Hutchins, E. (1997). *Screening for Substance Abuse During Pregnancy: Improving Care, Improving Health.* Arlington, VA: National Center for Education in Maternal and Child Health, Department of Health and Human Services.

Nassogne, M. C., Evrard, P., and Courtoy, P. J. (1998). Selective Direct Toxicity of Cocaine on Fetal Mouse Neurons. Teratogenic Implications of Neurite and Apoptotic Neuronal Loss. In J. A. Harvey and B. E. Kosofsky (eds.), *Cocaine: Effects on the Developing Brain* (pp. 51–68). New York: The New York Academy of Sciences.

National Institute on Drug Abuse (1996). *National Pregnancy and Health Survey: Drug Use Among Women Delivering Live Births: 1992* (NIH Publication 96–3819). Rockville, MD: Department of Health and Human Services.

Ockene, J. K. (1987). Smoking Intervention: The Expanding Role of the Physician. *American Journal of Public Health, 77,* pp. 782–783.

Olson, H. C., and Burgess, D. M. (1997). Early Intervention for Children Prenatally Exposed to Alcohol and Other Drugs. In M. J. Guralnick (ed.), *The Effectiveness of Early Intervention.* Baltimore, MD: Brookes.

Pederson, L. L. (1982). Compliance with Physician Advice to Quit Smoking: A Review of the Literature. *Preventive Medicine, 11,* pp. 71–84.

Rahdert, E. R., ed. (1996). *Treatment for Drug-Exposed Women and Their Children: Advances in Research Methodology.* NIDA Research Monograph, No. 166. Rockville, MD: National Institutes of Health.

Richardson, G. A. (1998). Prenatal Cocaine Exposure: A Longitudinal Study of Development. In J. A. Harvey and B. E. Kosofsky (eds.), *Cocaine: Effects on the Developing Brain* (pp. 144–152). New York: The New York Academy of Sciences.

Romano, A. G., and Harvey, J. A. (1998). Prenatal Cocaine Exposure: Long-Term Deficits in Learning and Motor Performance. In J. A. Harvey and B. E. Kosofsky (eds.), *Cocaine: Effects on the Developing Brain* (pp. 89–108). New York: The New York Academy of Sciences.

Rydell, C. P., and Everingham, S. S. (1994). *Controlling Cocaine: Supply vs. Demand Programs* (MR-331-ONDCP/A/DPRC). Santa Monica, CA: RAND. (Summary available in *Projecting Future Cocaine Use and Evaluating Control Strategies,* RAND Drug Policy Research Center Research Brief, RB–6002, January 1995.)

Santolaria-Fernandez, F. J., Gomez-Sirvent, J. L., Gonzalez-Reimers, C. E., Batista-Lopez, J. N., Jorge-Hernandez, J. A., Rodriguez-Moreno, F., Martinez-Riera, A., and Hernandez-Garcia, M. T.

(1995). Nutritional Assessment of Drug Addicts. *Drug and Alcohol Dependence, 38,* pp. 11–18.

Slotkin, T. (1998). Moderator, Round Table 2. Consensus on Postnatal Deficits: Comparability of Human and Animal Findings. In J. A. Harvey and B. E. Kosofsky (eds.), *Cocaine: Effects on the Developing Brain* (pp. 153–157). New York: The New York Academy of Sciences.

Spear, L. P., Campbell, J., Snyder, K., Silveri, M., and Katovic, N. (1998). Animal Behavior Models. Increased Sensitivity to Stressors and Other Environmental Experiences after Prenatal Cocaine Exposure. In J. A. Harvey and B. E. Kosofsky (eds.), *Cocaine: Effects on the Developing Brain* (pp. 76–88). New York: The New York Academy of Sciences.

Substance Abuse and Mental Health Services Administration (1999). *1998 National Household Survey on Drug Abuse.* Rockville, MD: SAMHSA Office of Applied Studies, U.S. Department of Health and Human Services.

Sullivan, E., and Fleming, M. A. (1997). *Guide to Substance Abuse Services for Primary Care Physicians.* Rockville, MD: Center for Substance Abuse Treatment.

U.S. General Accounting Office (1997). *Parental Substance Abuse: Implications for Children, the Child Welfare System, and Foster-Care Outcomes* (GAO/T-HEHS-98-40). Testimony before the Subcommittee on Human Resources, Committee on Ways and Means, House of Representatives.

Zellman, G. (1997). Health Care System Response to Prenatal Substance Exposure. Report to the National Institute on Drug Abuse (unpublished progress report prepared for internal use by NIDA).

Zellman, G., and Bell, R. (1990). *The Role of Professional Background, Case Characteristics, and Protective Agency Response in Mandated Child Abuse Reporting* (R-3825-HHS). Santa Monica, CA: RAND.

Zellman, G. L., Jacobson, P. D., and Bell, R. M. (1997). Influencing Physician Response to Prenatal Substance Exposure Through State Legislation and Work-Place Policies. *Addiction, 92,* pp. 1123–1131.

Zellman, G. L., Jacobson, P. D., DuPlessis, H., and DiMatteo, M. R. (1993). Detecting Prenatal Substance Exposure: An Exploratory Analysis and Policy Discussion. *Journal of Drug Issues, 23,* pp. 375–387.

Zellman, G. L., Jacobson, P. D., DuPlessis, H., and DiMatteo, M. R. (1992). *Health Care System Response to Prenatal Substance Use: An Exploratory Analysis.* Santa Monica, CA: RAND.

Suzanne L. Wenzel
RAND, Santa Monica, California

Barry E. Kosofsky
Massachusetts General Hospital and Harvard Medical School,
Boston, Massachusetts

John A. Harvey
MCP Hahnemann University, Philadelphia, Pennsylvania

Martin Y. Iguchi
RAND, Santa Monica, California

Paul Steinberg
RAND, Santa Monica, California

Katherine E. Watkins
RAND, Santa Monica, California

Rashid Shaikh
New York Academy of Sciences, New York, New York